TAPPING SOLUTION FOR WEIGHT LOSS

Journal

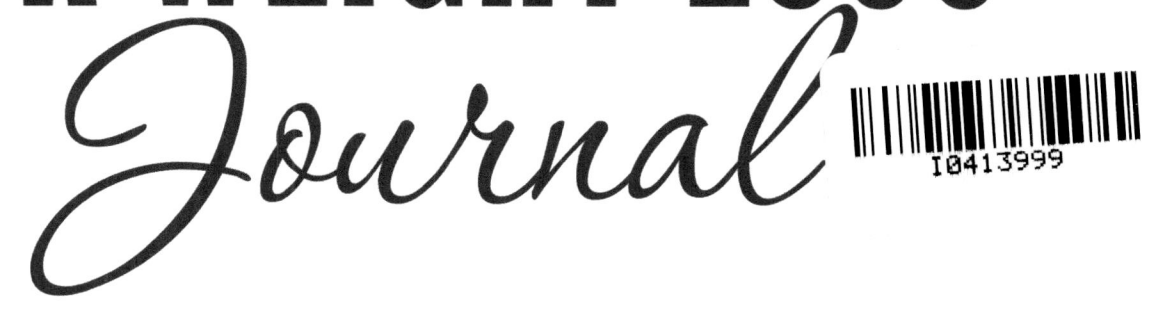

TRACK YOUR PROGRESS
SEE WHAT WORKS

A Must For Anyone On The

Tapping Solution for Weight Loss Diet

Speedy Publishing LLC
40 E. Main St. #1156
Newark, DE 19711

www.SpeedyPublishing.Com

Copyright 2014
978-1-63287-424-5
First Printed May 5, 2014

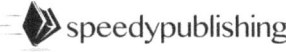

speedypublishing

Date _____   Weight _____

Feelings Before

_____

_____

_____

_____

_____

Location	
Phrase	
Location	
Phrase	
Location	
Phrase	
Location	
Phrase	
Location	
Phrase	
Location	
Phrase	
Location	
Phrase	

Feelings After

_____

_____

_____

_____

Date _____ Weight _____

Feelings Before

_____

_____

_____

_____

_____

Location	
Phrase	
Location	
Phrase	
Location	
Phrase	
Location	
Phrase	
Location	
Phrase	
Location	
Phrase	
Location	
Phrase	

Feelings After

_____

_____

_____

_____

_____

Date _____   Weight _____

Feelings Before

_____

_____

_____

_____

Location	
Phrase	
Location	
Phrase	
Location	
Phrase	
Location	
Phrase	
Location	
Phrase	
Location	
Phrase	
Location	
Phrase	

Feelings After

_____

_____

_____

_____

Date _____   Weight _____

Feelings Before

_____

_____

_____

_____

_____

Location	
Phrase	
Location	
Phrase	
Location	
Phrase	
Location	
Phrase	
Location	
Phrase	
Location	
Phrase	
Location	
Phrase	

Feelings After

_____

_____

_____

_____

Date _____   Weight _____

Feelings Before

_____
_____
_____
_____
_____

Location	
Phrase	
Location	
Phrase	
Location	
Phrase	
Location	
Phrase	
Location	
Phrase	
Location	
Phrase	
Location	
Phrase	

Feelings After

_____
_____
_____
_____
_____

Date _____ Weight _____

Feelings Before

_____
_____
_____
_____
_____

Location	
Phrase	
Location	
Phrase	
Location	
Phrase	
Location	
Phrase	
Location	
Phrase	
Location	
Phrase	
Location	
Phrase	

Feelings After

_____
_____
_____
_____
_____

Date _____ Weight _____

Feelings Before

_____

_____

_____

_____

_____

Location	
Phrase	
Location	
Phrase	
Location	
Phrase	
Location	
Phrase	
Location	
Phrase	
Location	
Phrase	
Location	
Phrase	

Feelings After

_____

_____

_____

_____

_____

Date _____   Weight _____

Feelings Before

_____

_____

_____

_____

_____

Location	
Phrase	
Location	
Phrase	
Location	
Phrase	
Location	
Phrase	
Location	
Phrase	
Location	
Phrase	
Location	
Phrase	

Feelings After

_____

_____

_____

_____

Date _____ Weight _____

Feelings Before

_____
_____
_____
_____
_____

Location	
Phrase	
Location	
Phrase	
Location	
Phrase	
Location	
Phrase	
Location	
Phrase	
Location	
Phrase	
Location	
Phrase	

Feelings After

_____
_____
_____
_____

Date _____   Weight _____

Feelings Before

_____
_____
_____
_____
_____

Location	
Phrase	
Location	
Phrase	
Location	
Phrase	
Location	
Phrase	
Location	
Phrase	
Location	
Phrase	
Location	
Phrase	

Feelings After

_____
_____
_____
_____
_____

Date _____   Weight _____

Feelings Before

_____
_____
_____
_____
_____

Location	
Phrase	
Location	
Phrase	
Location	
Phrase	
Location	
Phrase	
Location	
Phrase	
Location	
Phrase	
Location	
Phrase	

Feelings After

_____
_____
_____
_____
_____

Date _____   Weight _____

Feelings Before

_____
_____
_____
_____
_____

Location	
Phrase	
Location	
Phrase	
Location	
Phrase	
Location	
Phrase	
Location	
Phrase	
Location	
Phrase	
Location	
Phrase	

Feelings After

_____
_____
_____
_____
_____

Date _____   Weight _____

Feelings Before

_____
_____
_____
_____
_____

Location |
Phrase |
Location |
Phrase |
Location |
Phrase |
Location |
Phrase |
Location |
Phrase |
Location |
Phrase |
Location |
Phrase |

Feelings After

_____
_____
_____
_____
_____

Date _____ Weight _____

Feelings Before

_____
_____
_____
_____
_____

Location	
Phrase	
Location	
Phrase	
Location	
Phrase	
Location	
Phrase	
Location	
Phrase	
Location	
Phrase	
Location	
Phrase	

Feelings After

_____
_____
_____
_____
_____

Date _____   Weight _____

Feelings Before

_____

_____

_____

_____

_____

Location	
Phrase	
Location	
Phrase	
Location	
Phrase	
Location	
Phrase	
Location	
Phrase	
Location	
Phrase	
Location	
Phrase	

Feelings After

_____

_____

_____

_____

Date _____   Weight _____

Feelings Before

_____
_____
_____
_____
_____

Location	
Phrase	
Location	
Phrase	
Location	
Phrase	
Location	
Phrase	
Location	
Phrase	
Location	
Phrase	
Location	
Phrase	

Feelings After

_____
_____
_____
_____
_____

Date _____ Weight _____

Feelings Before

_____

_____

_____

_____

_____

Location	
Phrase	
Location	
Phrase	
Location	
Phrase	
Location	
Phrase	
Location	
Phrase	
Location	
Phrase	
Location	
Phrase	

Feelings After

_____

_____

_____

_____

Date _____ Weight _____

Feelings Before

_____
_____
_____
_____
_____

Location	
Phrase	
Location	
Phrase	
Location	
Phrase	
Location	
Phrase	
Location	
Phrase	
Location	
Phrase	
Location	
Phrase	

Feelings After

_____
_____
_____
_____
_____

Date _____   Weight _____

Feelings Before

_____

_____

_____

_____

_____

Location	
Phrase	
Location	
Phrase	
Location	
Phrase	
Location	
Phrase	
Location	
Phrase	
Location	
Phrase	
Location	
Phrase	

Feelings After

_____

_____

_____

_____

_____

Date _____ Weight _____

Feelings Before

_____

_____

_____

_____

_____

Location	
Phrase	
Location	
Phrase	
Location	
Phrase	
Location	
Phrase	
Location	
Phrase	
Location	
Phrase	
Location	
Phrase	

Feelings After

_____

_____

_____

_____

Date _____   Weight _____

Feelings Before

_____
_____
_____
_____
_____

Location	
Phrase	
Location	
Phrase	
Location	
Phrase	
Location	
Phrase	
Location	
Phrase	
Location	
Phrase	
Location	
Phrase	

Feelings After

_____
_____
_____
_____
_____

Date _____   Weight _____

Feelings Before

_____
_____
_____
_____
_____

Location | _____
Phrase | _____
Location | _____
Phrase | _____
Location | _____
Phrase | _____
Location | _____
Phrase | _____
Location | _____
Phrase | _____
Location | _____
Phrase | _____
Location | _____
Phrase | _____

Feelings After

_____
_____
_____
_____
_____

Date _____   Weight _____

Feelings Before

_____

_____

_____

_____

_____

Location	
Phrase	
Location	
Phrase	
Location	
Phrase	
Location	
Phrase	
Location	
Phrase	
Location	
Phrase	
Location	
Phrase	

Feelings After

_____

_____

_____

_____

Date _____   Weight _____

Feelings Before

_____
_____
_____
_____
_____

Location	
Phrase	
Location	
Phrase	
Location	
Phrase	
Location	
Phrase	
Location	
Phrase	
Location	
Phrase	
Location	
Phrase	

Feelings After

_____
_____
_____
_____
_____

Date _____   Weight _____

Feelings Before

_____
_____
_____
_____
_____

Location	
Phrase	
Location	
Phrase	
Location	
Phrase	
Location	
Phrase	
Location	
Phrase	
Location	
Phrase	
Location	
Phrase	

Feelings After

_____
_____
_____
_____
_____

Date _____ Weight _____

Feelings Before

_____

_____

_____

_____

_____

Location	
Phrase	
Location	
Phrase	
Location	
Phrase	
Location	
Phrase	
Location	
Phrase	
Location	
Phrase	
Location	
Phrase	

Feelings After

_____

_____

_____

_____

_____

Date _____ Weight _____

Feelings Before

_____

_____

_____

_____

_____

Location	
Phrase	
Location	
Phrase	
Location	
Phrase	
Location	
Phrase	
Location	
Phrase	
Location	
Phrase	
Location	
Phrase	

Feelings After

_____

_____

_____

_____

Date _____   Weight _____

Feelings Before

_____
_____
_____
_____
_____

Location	
Phrase	
Location	
Phrase	
Location	
Phrase	
Location	
Phrase	
Location	
Phrase	
Location	
Phrase	
Location	
Phrase	

Feelings After

_____
_____
_____
_____
_____

Date _____ Weight _____

Feelings Before

_____
_____
_____
_____
_____

Location	
Phrase	
Location	
Phrase	
Location	
Phrase	
Location	
Phrase	
Location	
Phrase	
Location	
Phrase	
Location	
Phrase	

Feelings After

_____
_____
_____
_____

Date _____   Weight _____

Feelings Before

_____
_____
_____
_____
_____

Location	
Phrase	
Location	
Phrase	
Location	
Phrase	
Location	
Phrase	
Location	
Phrase	
Location	
Phrase	
Location	
Phrase	

Feelings After

_____
_____
_____
_____

Date _____ Weight _____

Feelings Before

_____
_____
_____
_____
_____

Location	
Phrase	
Location	
Phrase	
Location	
Phrase	
Location	
Phrase	
Location	
Phrase	
Location	
Phrase	
Location	
Phrase	

Feelings After

_____
_____
_____
_____
_____

Date _____   Weight _____

Feelings Before

_____

_____

_____

_____

_____

Location	
Phrase	
Location	
Phrase	
Location	
Phrase	
Location	
Phrase	
Location	
Phrase	
Location	
Phrase	
Location	
Phrase	

Feelings After

_____

_____

_____

_____

_____

Date _____ Weight _____

Feelings Before

_____

_____

_____

_____

_____

Location	
Phrase	
Location	
Phrase	
Location	
Phrase	
Location	
Phrase	
Location	
Phrase	
Location	
Phrase	
Location	
Phrase	

Feelings After

_____

_____

_____

_____

_____

Date _____ Weight _____

Feelings Before

_____

_____

_____

_____

_____

Location	
Phrase	
Location	
Phrase	
Location	
Phrase	
Location	
Phrase	
Location	
Phrase	
Location	
Phrase	
Location	
Phrase	

Feelings After

_____

_____

_____

_____

Date _____   Weight _____

Feelings Before

_____

_____

_____

_____

_____

Location	
Phrase	
Location	
Phrase	
Location	
Phrase	
Location	
Phrase	
Location	
Phrase	
Location	
Phrase	
Location	
Phrase	
Location	
Phrase	

Feelings After

_____

_____

_____

_____

Date _____   Weight _____

Feelings Before

_____
_____
_____
_____
_____

Location	
Phrase	
Location	
Phrase	
Location	
Phrase	
Location	
Phrase	
Location	
Phrase	
Location	
Phrase	
Location	
Phrase	

Feelings After

_____
_____
_____
_____

Date _____   Weight _____

Feelings Before

_____

_____

_____

_____

_____

Location	
Phrase	
Location	
Phrase	
Location	
Phrase	
Location	
Phrase	
Location	
Phrase	
Location	
Phrase	
Location	
Phrase	

Feelings After

_____

_____

_____

_____

_____

Date _____   Weight _____

Feelings Before

_____

_____

_____

_____

_____

Location	
Phrase	
Location	
Phrase	
Location	
Phrase	
Location	
Phrase	
Location	
Phrase	
Location	
Phrase	
Location	
Phrase	

Feelings After

_____

_____

_____

_____

Date _____   Weight _____

Feelings Before

_____

_____

_____

_____

_____

Location	
Phrase	
Location	
Phrase	
Location	
Phrase	
Location	
Phrase	
Location	
Phrase	
Location	
Phrase	
Location	
Phrase	

Feelings After

_____

_____

_____

_____

Date _____   Weight _____

Feelings Before

_____
_____
_____
_____
_____

Location	
Phrase	
Location	
Phrase	
Location	
Phrase	
Location	
Phrase	
Location	
Phrase	
Location	
Phrase	
Location	
Phrase	

Feelings After

_____
_____
_____
_____
_____

Date _____ Weight _____

Feelings Before

_____
_____
_____
_____
_____

Location	
Phrase	
Location	
Phrase	
Location	
Phrase	
Location	
Phrase	
Location	
Phrase	
Location	
Phrase	
Location	
Phrase	

Feelings After

_____
_____
_____
_____

Date _____ Weight _____

Feelings Before

_____

_____

_____

_____

_____

Location	
Phrase	
Location	
Phrase	
Location	
Phrase	
Location	
Phrase	
Location	
Phrase	
Location	
Phrase	
Location	
Phrase	

Feelings After

_____

_____

_____

_____

_____

Date _____   Weight _____

Feelings Before

_____

_____

_____

_____

_____

Location	
Phrase	
Location	
Phrase	
Location	
Phrase	
Location	
Phrase	
Location	
Phrase	
Location	
Phrase	
Location	
Phrase	

Feelings After

_____

_____

_____

_____

_____

Date _____   Weight _____

Feelings Before

_____

_____

_____

_____

_____

Location	
Phrase	
Location	
Phrase	
Location	
Phrase	
Location	
Phrase	
Location	
Phrase	
Location	
Phrase	
Location	
Phrase	

Feelings After

_____

_____

_____

_____

Date _____ Weight _____

Feelings Before

_____
_____
_____
_____
_____

Location	
Phrase	
Location	
Phrase	
Location	
Phrase	
Location	
Phrase	
Location	
Phrase	
Location	
Phrase	
Location	
Phrase	

Feelings After

_____
_____
_____
_____

Date _____ Weight _____

Feelings Before

_____
_____
_____
_____
_____

Location	
Phrase	
Location	
Phrase	
Location	
Phrase	
Location	
Phrase	
Location	
Phrase	
Location	
Phrase	
Location	
Phrase	

Feelings After

_____
_____
_____
_____

Date _____   Weight _____

Feelings Before

_____
_____
_____
_____
_____

Location	
Phrase	
Location	
Phrase	
Location	
Phrase	
Location	
Phrase	
Location	
Phrase	
Location	
Phrase	
Location	
Phrase	

Feelings After

_____
_____
_____
_____
_____

Date _____ Weight _____

Feelings Before

_____

_____

_____

_____

_____

Location	
Phrase	
Location	
Phrase	
Location	
Phrase	
Location	
Phrase	
Location	
Phrase	
Location	
Phrase	
Location	
Phrase	

Feelings After

_____

_____

_____

_____

_____